I0789306

The Medeic Body Type

Representing one of the 22 Body Types first described by Victor Rocine around 1900

The Gary Oldman, Madonna Celebrity Body Type

For Kaye,
there at the beginning with Doc Severn,
and for Liberty,
continuing the holistic healing journey…

———

About the Author

Educated in New Zealand and in the U.S.A., Dr. Stenbeck attained B.Sc. (NZ), M.S., and D.C. degrees. His holistic healing methods have been profiled in magazines (Esquire, McLean's, Playgirl, the Atlanta Constitution), and on TV in the USA and in Canada. He was the main contributor to the Warner Book, _The Eye/Body Connection_ by Jessica Maxwell that focused on the holistic healing relationships between the iris structure and organ genetics.

In the 1970-80's he was elected Fellow, Royal Society of Health, London; Fellow, American Association of Chemists; Member, American Association of Clinical Chemists; and Affiliate, Royal Society of Medicine, London. He studied naturopathy and Body Types with Dr. Bernard Jensen and Dr. Clifford Severn, and has practiced in medical partnerships where patients received the joint benefits of medical and holistic healing.

He is a member of Self-Realization Fellowship. To receive advice on any health issue from a holistic viewpoint, or to receive help with your body type, see his web site: *DrStenbeck.net*

———

Contents

* * *

The Medeic Body Type and Food Guide   *1*

<u>*Appendix*</u>

The 22 Body Types:
Celebrity Examples

This Booklet contains the Pargenic type. See <u>The 22 Unique Body Types</u> for all type descript-ions.]

Thin Types

Atrophic	*Woody Allen / Audrey Hepburn* *Stan Laurel / Calista Flockheart*
Exesthesic	*Cher / Sarah Jessica Parker* *(Female type only)*
Marasmic	*President Obama / Princess Diana* *James Stewart / Kate Blanchard*
Neurogenic	*J.K. Simmons / Joan Rivers* *Jon Cryer / Marin Hinle*
Pathoferic	*(No celebrity males)* *Blythe Danner / Gwyneth Paltrow*
Sillevitic	*David Bowie / Shirley MacLaine* *Rod Stewart / Carol Channing*

Muscle Types

Calciferic   *Michael Jordan / Angelica Huston*
          Abraham Lincoln / Grace Jones

Carbogenic   *George Clooney / Lady Gaga*
          Pres. G. Bush, Jr. / Meg Ryan

Desmogenic   *Marlon Brando / Loni Anderson*
          Daniel Craig / Tina Turner

Eldic   *Ross Perot / Hillary Clinton*
          Peter Falk / Sigourney Weaver

Medeic   *Gary Oldman, Madonna*

Myogenic   *Pres. Bill Clinton / Sharon Stone*
          Pres. John Kennedy / Julia Roberts

Nervimotive   *Frank Sinatra / Elizabeth Taylor*
          Mark Wahlberg / Natalie Wood

Nitropheric   *Ben Affleck / Ava Gardner*
          Kirk Douglas / Kate Winslet

Pallinomic   *Pres. Donald Trump /*
          Attorney General Janet Reno
          Bill O'Reilly (Fox) / Jane Russell

Fat Types

Barotic   Robin Williams / 'Mrs.Doubtfire'
          Elton John / William Conrad

Carboferic   Bill Murray / Roseanne
             Billy Gardell / Melissa McCarthy

Hydripheric   John Goodman / Shelly Winters
              Wayne Knight / Jennifer Holliday

Isogenic   Einstein / Oprah Winfrey
           Phillip S .Hoffman / Queen Victoria

Lipopheric   Rush Limbaugh / Rosie O'Donnell
             Chris Christie / Camryn Manheim

Oxypheric   Winston Churchill / Orsen Welles
            Ella Fitzgerald / Gerry Spence

Pargenic   Burt Reynolds / Katey Segal
           Ron Perlman / Kirstey Alley

Dr.Lloyd Stenbeck

<u>*Succinct Quote on Human Types*</u>

From Victor Rocine, who first described discrete body types around 1900.

"A type is an order of people that differentiates and distinguishes itself by a general and similar form, brain-formation, chemistry, structure, build, immunity, tendencies, predisposition, resemblance, skin-pigment, and type characteristics based on observation and analogy.

"Or, in other words, people of a given type are similar physically and like-minded as if they were brothers and sisters—that is what type means.

"Everything in nature is made according to plan. Man only discovers that plan and gives it a name. The zoologist has not made the animals—he has only described the plan adopted by the wonderful Creator, and named the classes, sub-classes, etc.

"How important type research will be to humanity, time alone will make known."

———

Prologue

The esteemed scientist J. J. Berzelius, discoverer of several chemical elements, inspired Victor Rocine to research body types and to investigate the correlation between types and their diseases. Around 1890-1910, Rocine privately published his original findings on the mineral basis of different body types, and this present book exists because of his brilliant insights.

For many years, I studied with Dr. Clifford Severn who had been a personal student of Victor Rocine on body types, naturopathy, herbology, iris analysis, diet, and nutritional healing methods. He had a successful career as a lecturer and healer, and was one of those rare athletes with complete muscle control over his body. I saw him under a spotlight at 85 years of age, contracting and rippling every individual muscle in his perfectly developed body. Field-Marshal Jan Smuts, the WWII South African Prime Minister, devoted a full chapter of his autobiography to how Severn's healing methods had saved his life. In the 1950's, *Life* magazine did a four-page spread on Severn and his family. Fame he had.

Another Rocine student I studied with, Dr. Bernard Jensen wrote of Rocine's body type research and nutritional methods in his privately published, *The Chemistry of Man*.

This book is deeply rooted in Rocine's original work, and with that of Herbert Shelton, M.D., Ph.D. (at Harvard University in the 1930's). I integrated their research with newer dietary and nervous system data along with celebrity examples of each type, hopefully, making this material easier to digest and more entertaining for the reader.

Gayelord Hauser, another Rocine student I knew, was a celebrated health book author. He wrote a popular book on Rocine's types in the 1940's, *Types and Temperaments;* reputedly, he also introduced yogurt to the western world.

This book exists because of Rocine's creative brilliance and original discoveries in natural healing.

▶ *Rocine: "The soul creates the body type."*

Rocine taught that the soul chooses a body type and brain to live in, thus presenting different experiences and life lessons to master. Why were *you* born the way you are?

That is something to think about, especially if it is true! What would your soul purpose be to live in a particular body type. I provide some thoughts on this issue in each type description and try to assess from my experience with your type the particular lessons of life presented therein.

Rocine was as brilliant in his way as an Abraham Lincoln, Michael Jordan, Michael Phelps, Tony Robbins, or a Daniel Day Lewis—all *calciferic* types—rare, leaders, innovative, brilliant, and highly intelligent in their different fields of endeavor.

Celebrity examples exist for most types, not a duplicate of you, but someone who has your essence in their body-mind individuality. Knowing your type allows you to become a better you!

The celebrity examples provide further help in identifying your body type.

► *Rocine's classic findings, the backbone of this book, are integrated with Sheldon's research and with other dietary and food issues including mental, emotional, and spiritual attributes,*

Many people take nutritional supplements and try different diets without a doctor's advice. If this is your choice, use common sense, listen to body responses, and discontinue any allergic reactions to foods or nutritional substances.

———

The Medeic Body Type

"You may also have a physical or psychological feature not representative of your type such as height, weight, appearance, talent, weakness, strength, etc., due to biochemical errors, environmental influences, racial or cultural differences and congenital or genetic issues. Nevertheless, the type identification of the average person is usually clear."

—Victor Rocine

Medeic Type Celebrity Examples

*If you think this is your type, be sure to look at **<u>on-line photographs</u>** of these examples. Look for general similarities to yourself. Note that sub-types cause the differences in appearance between members of the same type. This is a relatively rare body type.*

————

ACTORS

David Caruso (CSI: Miami)
Gary Oldman
Humphrey Bogart
Henry Silva
Steve Buscemi
Marlene Dietrich
Sarah Bernhardt (classic actor)

VOICE/MUSIC

Mick Jagger
Keith Richards
Charlie Watts
(Three 'Rolling Stones' and other rock star members are this type.)

Madonna
Sandra Bernhard

SPORTS

Cesar Chavez (And many light-weight boxers)

OTHER

Rev. Jim Bakker
Diamanda Galas (singer)
Tim Burton (director)

HISTORICAL (From Rocine)

Nietzsche
Dante
Edgar Allan Poe
Robespierre
Paderewski
Voltaire
Richard III
Jesse James

And
Duchess Wallis Simpson (wife of King Edward VIII)

[Note: I have known several members of this type, and others in everyday life, which contributed to my understanding of the type.]

You already know something about this type from their public persona and appearance, whether from seeing them yourself or from the celebrity examples. Blend such insights with the type descriptions and the types of your family and friends to discern their presence in your midst!

Read the types, and if still confused you may choose to use the personal request for type identification from my web site: *DrStenbeck.net*

———

Medeic Type Questionnaire

These questions describe the generic type, and not specifically you! If any question ever applied to you, then choose the True answer!

For Question 1 only:

A = True	B = Maybe	C = Untrue
15 points	7 points	1 point

1. Physically identify with celebrity example ____

Then...

A = True	B = Maybe	C = Untrue
5 points	3 points	1 point

---

2. Height is close to:
   Males: 5'4-5'9   Females: 5'0-5'8   ____
3. Usual weight is close to:
   Males: 120-165   Females: 85-155   ____
4. Body usually lean, gaunt, slender,
   rugged, wiry in appearance   ____
5. Muscles small, compact, strong; body
   taut, muscular   ____
6. Weight easily controlled; difficult to
   gain weight   ____
7. May smoke cigarettes (or used to)   ____
8. Dark, black, stiff hair   ____

9. Bold cheek bones, sunken cheeks,
    darker complexion   _____
10. Easily brought to anger or rage   _____
11. Strong sexual drive, highly sexual
    and sensual from an early age   _____
12. Teeth strong, may be malformed,
    discolored, or odd-sized   _____
13 May be overly-familiar, or antisocial _____
14. Able to weight-lift, are strong   _____
15. Mostly have a plain appearance   _____
16. Male chest and body has little hair;
    bust usually small to medium-sized   _____
17. Very cautious and conscientious   _____
18. Gesticulate when talking   _____
19. Have a long memory for hurts   _____
20. Lips may be overly red, atypical, thin;
    may crack; lower lip often darker   _____
21. If offended, are quick to punish   _____
22. May be disrespectful   _____
23. Tend to live in past memories   _____
24. Lack faith, trust, hope   _____
25. Overly-active memory for prior
    bad experiences   _____
26. May look unhappy and foreboding   _____
27. May use or abuse alcohol or drugs   _____
28. Highly developed sense of justice   _____
29. May look older than you are   _____
30. May feel revengeful   _____
31. Darker complexion, serious or
    threatening appearance (without
    meaning to be that way)   _____

32. Brown, blue eyes typical; eyes may be
smaller than average; eyebrows bushy _____
33. Smaller, irregular ears (mostly males) _____
34. Nose large or small and squat;
nose-tip may be long _____
35. Face square or square-circular with
angular features _____
36. Mouth medium-sized or smaller;
mouth may droop _____
37. Strong teeth and gums (some irregular)_____
38. Mind tends to be negative _____
39. Have strongly developed muscles;
body is tough; difficult for foes to
defeat or conquer you _____
40. Hair often grays early _____
41. Flat strong back; shoulders broad,
bony and strong _____
42. Hips, abdomen flat; hollowed-in
stomach; no pot-belly _____
43. Deep voice, low-pitched, forceful,
plain-speaking, insistent, authoritative,
commanding _____
44. Long extremities (may look awkward);
arms stronger than legs; may have
beak-like nails _____
45. Tend to be unhappy and worried _____
46. May be a troubled child: breaking
windows, sexually active, stealing,
school expulsions, etc. _____
47. May be anti-social when young _____
48. Do things to excess; either too liberal
or too strict _____

49. May have oratorical, inspiring ability   _____
50. Have a dramatic personality   _____
51. May have intuitive, clairvoyant ability   _____
52. Originality in your area of expertise is
     a leading trait   _____
53. Very clever and may be brilliant   _____
54. May need therapy   _____
55. May walk around talking to yourself   _____
56. Have great tenacity   _____
57. Very excitable and restless   _____
58. Usually polite and congenial; some
     are opinionated, sarcastic   _____
59. Defend self with fists or speech;
     are ready to fight to the death   _____
60. Plain or attractive face, curved
     cheekbones, the lower jaw is long   _____
61. Are great lovers of music; musical
     talents (many rock performers)   _____
62. Impatient; easily lose control   _____
63. Some have a dark-side (and be
     profane, insolent, suspicious)   _____

Scoring

For Question #1:

A response: give 15 points = ________
   B response: give 7 points = ________
   C response: give 1 points = ________

For Questions #2—63:

   A response: give 5 points = ________
   B response: give 3 points = ________
   C response: give 1 point = ________

Total of the above points = ________

Interpretation

158—295: PROBABLY Medeic type

85—157: POSSIBLY Medeic type

<85: NOT Medeic type

The Medeic Type

Rocine: "Medeic means 'the holding of toxins' resulting in unhealthy physical, mental and emotional states." You are a <u>potassium, calcium, and phosphorus</u> type. You are potentially brilliant, with an acute sense of drama and tragedy.

You are humorous, spiritual, loyal, sexual, sensuous, strong, and rebellious. When younger your lean or wiry body is gaunt and you may look like a thin type; for example, David Caruso (CSI Miami), Madonna, Mick Jagger of the Rolling Stones, and Humphrey Bogart—lean, strong, and ruggedly handsome or attractive. You are a rare type.

▶ *Rocine: "You tend to be fixated with sexual behavior and may become sexually addicted; when younger, help may be needed to understand and moderate this 'genetic addiction.' You need a mate who shares your sexual cravings. Substance abuse is common in the medeic: nicotine, pot, drugs, and/or alcohol. God is your salvation."*

[Written around 1900, Rocine had bias about this type, and his comments are not necessarily true today, although it fits some of you.]

Madonna has the *medeic* behavioral aspects down pat! Her liberated sexual values and behaviors are familiar to us all. She probably has a sub-type giving her a more medium-build; yet, there are younger photos clearly showing her sinewy, lean, and muscular body. The great movie star Marlene Deitrich was lean, sexual, innovative, challenging, stern, and commandingly self-assured. Mick Jagger and many hard rock singers have that lean gaunt look, but are as strong as lions. The immortal classical tragic actor, Sarah Bernhardt, from the early 1900's is another typical example.

———

Physical Similarity to Other Types

The *nervimotive* type (Frank Sinatra, Elizabeth Taylor) is somewhat similar, expressive, and usually more attractive.

The *neurogenic* type (J. J. Simmons, Joan Rivers) is often lean when younger, and is more friendly and approachable.

The *sillevitic* type (David Bowie, Florence Henderson) is more happy, optimistic and outgoing.

———

Average Height and Weight

Males:	5'4-5'9	120-165 pounds
Females:	5'0-5'8	85-155 pounds

———

Medeic Type Description

The type description represents how you appear in everyday society. You may have a sub-type that alters parts of this description.

Think of the celebrity examples as you read the descriptions. You are lean to medium-sized, and may look older than you are. Some of you look haggard and stoop-shouldered.

Head — Your head, face and forehead are square or rectangular shaped. The head movements are usually jerky.

Hair — Your hair is dark or black, with some brunettes, and is usually bushy and strong. You tend to turn gray at an early age, often by age 30.

Eyes — Darker or blue eyes, smaller then average, are characteristic; the eyebrows are bushy, dark. You complain of eye spots, flashes and pains.

Ears — Small and irregular shaped ears are common.

Nose — Your nose is often small and squat, occasionally larger; the nose-tip may be long.

Face — You have a square or rectangular face on frontal view. The face is angular and not necessarily smooth: acne or pock-marks are common (predominantly in males, and also seen in the *pargenic and desmogenic*). Marked cheekbones, sunken cheeks, and a large upper jaw are usual.

Mouth and Lips — Your mouth is small to medium-sized, with thin lips vulnerable to cracking: note the lips of Rev. Jim Bakker and David Caruso. Your voice is deep, forceful, insistent, demanding, authoritative, low-pitched, and plain speaking: people pay attention to you!

▶ *I have observed that you may curl the upper lip and talk through the corner of your mouth. Some of you have an unusual lip shape, color, congestion, or other irregularity.*

Teeth — Your teeth and gums are typically strong, sometimes irregular.

Skin — The skin is tough, tending to age and wrinkle with a leathery appearance. Darker hues may occur in the skin, with freckles, moles, acne, scarring, and other imperfections.

Nose — A long and wiry neck is usual.

Muscles — Potassium gives you a powerful musculature, the body being wiry, rugged, and tough.

Chest — The male chest is flat, little hair; the bust is usually small or medium-sized.

Back and Shoulders — A flat and strong back is usual; the shoulders are broad, bony, strong, and tapering to the feet; some stoop-shoul-dered.

Hips and Abdomen — Your hips are flat and thin, and hollowed in at the stomach. The abdomen is flat in both sexes—you do not get a pot-belly.

Arms and Legs — You have long extremities, hands and feet, and may look awkward. Your arms may be stronger than your legs, and you gesticulate when talking. You may have "beak-like" finger nails.

Joints — Strong, dense, elastic, normal-sized bones and joints are typical.

———

Medeic Personality Traits

If you are this type many, but not all, of the following characteristics are present—you may have overcome or moderated the negatives, but recognize that you once had several of them.

You may have any of the following traits:

- Have very active hand gestures
- Are dramatic, may be awe-inspiring
- Readily defend self with speech or fists
- Are assertive or aggressive, never passive
- Have only a few close and trusted friends
- Are very able to defend yourself in speech
- Highly developed satirical sense of humor
- Excitable, sociable, talkative (when healthy)
- Your feelings may be affectionate, or hateful
- Prefer heat: baths, showers, drinks, foods, etc.

- Usually are polite, congenial (some are negative)

▶ *Rocine: "You are original, inventive, innovative, and often brilliant or a genius."*

- Great lovers of rock music, may have musical talents
- May follow an unorthodox religion or spiritual direction
- May be intuitive or clairvoyant; are quick to condemn evil
- When in a positive mental state, may adopt special diets and nutritional support for health.
- Admire power and destructiveness: are attracted to the police and military and are excellent soldiers
- You tend to have oratorical powers, and the ability to stimulate and inspire people (e.g., Rev. Jim Bakker).
- Are tenacious, not easily defeated: you may fight to the death (like the *carbogenic, desmogenic, and nervimotive* types).

▶ *On a TV show, I heard Orsen Welles say about his medeic wife Marlene Deitrich: "She was a ferociously loyal person!" Once friendship is given, you are very loyal.*

———

Potential Challenges

You may have evolved from, or not experienced these general faults, so don't dwell on them.

▶ *Rocine: "You take pride in your sexual prowess and sexuality, and believe there is no purity in humanity. Your type shows the extremes of the human condition from genius and enviable success, to drug addiction."*

- May need to be more social
- You may appear to be saintly, or not
- Are disrespectful and overly-familiar
- Very impatient, may easily lose control
- Tend to be troubled, unhappy, worried
- An intense sexual drive may cause trouble
- May be tempted or drawn into crime when young
- High-tempered, brazen, distrustful, and revengeful

- You always expect the worse, and tend to hold grudges
- Tend to do things to excess, either too liberal or too strict
- Some of you walk around talking to yourself; males may do this to a distraction.
- Some are sociopathic (church and parental support helps with adjusting to the societal norm)

▶ *Rocine, a calciferic type, one hundred years ago was very critical and biased about this type so don't take his negative comments too personally!*

- As children some of you may break windows, insult, steal, hurt people, kill animals, cut school, etc.
- Vulnerable to negative or morbid thinking: such thoughts may be moderated through therapy
- As teenagers some may be so troubled by sexual and anti-social passions that they become nuns or priests

———

Medeic Stress Management

You have strong *mental* stress prevention providing a good ability not to internalize this stress into your stomach, adrenals, and immune system. You are vulnerable to *emotional* stress, and any of the above challenges may need reprogramming help. *[If needing help managing these stresses, see my prior books.]*

Love

In love relationships you prefer people who defer to your considerable sexual demands; you are usually attracted to the *carboferic, carbogenic, and desmogenic* types.

Talents and Vocations

Abilities - *Military, police, chemistry, law, arts, singing, sales, inventing, religion, music, accounting, motivating others*

Many of you lack compassion and patience. You may be brilliant performers, writers, artists, actors, actors, and business people. The *medeic* people I have known are all positive, interesting, and loving, with common goals to be healthier and productive. The geniuses of your type are morbid, gloomy, and satirical.

▶ *I have known you as: writers, dancers, singers, accountants, actors, secretaries, and rock musicians. You have acting and speaking skills that if developed captivate others: you may be a spell-binding speaker (or singer).*

The type information cannot predict what or who you will become, but you are capable of bringing a creative excellence or brilliance to whatever you do in life.

Inabilities - *Humanitarian pursuits, detailed science*

You have little talent for work requiring compassion for others.

———

Health Problems

You tend to age early. When sick you experience health problems or diseases in these organs or tissues:

Central Nervous System — Brain and spinal cord toxicity from environmental pollution is common.

Heart — Your heart is vulnerable to stress and fatty infiltration; you need preventive health care.

Gastro-intestinal Tract — Ulcers, diverticulitis, colitis are common; you often have bad or sour breath.

Chronic Diseases — Chronic problems occur in membranes, muscles, cysts, and joints (arthritis).

Other — You may have peculiar throat sensations.

▶ *Rocine: "Drugs sabotage your health; you need to be with a nutritional doctor. Natural medicine is your savior."*

———

Medeic Acid/Alkaline Factor

[See Chapter 3 for details on this subject, along with the common symptoms found with people of different nervous system dominance.]

For your health and healing, the genetics of your autonomic nervous system predispose you to needing a specific ratio of food acidity to alkalinity. You are born with an **intermediate** constitution, which means you need a balance between acid and alkaline-ash foods in your diet. (Ash refers to the minerals left in your body after metabolizing foods.)

Your autonomic nervous system genetics are intermediate between the *parasympathetic* and *sympathetic* nervous systems, making this acid/alkaline question less important for you compared to the predominantly acid and alkaline types. Construct this *approximate* ratio of daily food selections:

> *50% Fruits, salads, vegetables*
> *50% Proteins, carbohydrates*

▶ *Approximate your food ratios. On any particular day, it does not matter if one meal is mostly alkaline and another mostly acid—just try to balance it out for the day! If you make a mistake, try again tomorrow. It is a subjective call that you make, as what you do over weeks and months makes the difference to your health.*

* * *

The Medeic Spiritual Factor

Skip this paragraph if uninterested in a philosophical perspective on your type!

If as souls, we choose the brain and body type to spend a lifetime in, it could be to learn certain spiritual lessons related to perfecting ourselves, and our humanity, in God's eyes. What lessons does the type bring you? Only you can really decide what those lessons are. You know your weaknesses, what goes through your mind, and behaviors towards others. You know things about yourself that Victor Rocine could never get from his research subjects when he first wrote about types. So search your mind for the answers.

▶ *Rocine: "The soul chooses the body type."*

Each discrete type has challenges of life lessons, spiritual goals, etc., and some of yours may be:

God-like? — Some of you think so! Consider that you are no better, or worse, than anyone else.

Morbid Thinking — You tend to expect the worst to happen in all important areas of your life; counseling helps resolve this issue. Your morbid thinking particularly needs assistance with mental body nutrition (calcium, phosphorus, B-complex) and positive affirmations.

Anti-social — You care little for societal rules, so give yourself permission to conform a little! The males may be vulnerable to crime when young; therapy and religion helps with socialization.

▶ *Rocine: "You may appear threatening to others."*

Destructiveness — An important weakness, particularly in males; as a child you need parental direction into boxing, contact sports, and religion!

Lack of Spiritual Faith — You may have low faith; parental action helps inspire you to have faith, although many of you never connect with God.

▶ *Rocine: "You need religion in your life."*

———

A Medeic Story...

Keith, age 34, an accountant, suffered from constipation, nervousness, headaches, and a morbid imagination; he was medically negative for disease. He was semi-vegetarian, appropriate for his type, but he had a phosphorus food deficit in his diet and needed daily: cheese, almonds, pinto beans, sunflower seeds, wheat breads, and soda water. He also showed a deficient intake of calcium and potassium foods: kelp, turnip greens, parsley, corn tortillas, watercress, tofu, and yogurt.

Keith's morbid imagination directly related to his body type genetics, exaggerated by his dietary problems. After making the necessary dietary changes his symptoms started resolving almost immediately.

———

Medeic Type Mineral Foods

Apply this mineral data to the diet following these Muscle type descriptions.

Excessive Foods:
- *Chlorine (salt, salted junk foods)*
- *Nitrogen (beef)*

Deficient Foods:
- *Phosphorus*
- *Potassium*
- *Calcium*
- *Fluorine*
- *Nitrogen (non-beef, vegetable)*

These deficient nutrients are common deficiencies in your type, and predispose you to ill-health.

If ill, be sure to use these lists with your <u>daily</u> food intake.

If not ill, eat from the foods lists 3-4 times <u>weekly</u>.

All food lists are in descending order of concentration and value to you; choose servings of foods in the upper half of each list first!

One serving is ½ cup.

Medeic Excessive Foods -

Chlorine from salted junk foods and the salt shaker is excessive in your type; avoid them as they contribute to your aging and to negative mental and emotional states.

Nitrogen from red meat is excessive in your diet (if eaten more than once weekly), and is a major cause of your acidity and illnesses; poultry, fish and eggs should be taken about four days weekly; eat vegetarian proteins like legumes (peas, beans), seeds, nuts and pasta on other days.

———

Deficient Foods -

In illness or disease, it is important to correct these deficiencies.

Phosphorus is often deficient and needed because of your intense nervous system activity and brain exhaustion. You are always thinking and worrying about everything in your life—especially your health.

Potassium is usually deficient in your type. It is concentrated in and vital to the health of your muscles, heart, brain, and all cells. If ill or diseased, potassium foods and supplements are probably a significant healing factor.

Calcium is usually deficient in your type. It is highly concentrated in bones, joints, muscles, nerves, heart, teeth, and gums; if you have an illness or disease in any of these tissues calcium foods and supplements may be a significant healing factor.

Fluorine is deficient in your type, and also in the *pargenic*. It is an essential component of connective tissues (teeth, gums, bones, joints, hair), and has an important anti-cavity and antiseptic healing function in the body.

Nitrogen from vegetable sources is deficient (see above note).

———

<u>Minimize</u>
Excessive Foods

Chlorine (salted, junk foods):
0-2 times/<u>week</u>

Salt, all fast foods, packaged foods, canned and frozen foods, soy sauce, all preserved meats (cured, smoked, canned and luncheon meats), sauces (barbecue, catsup, etc.), dill pickles, sauerkraut, bouillon cubes, peanut butter, potato chips, etc., salted nuts, crackers, canned or packaged soups, processed cheeses, commercial salad dressings, meat tenderizers.

Note: If you must eat anything on the above list, keep it down to 0-2 times weekly!

Nitrogen (animal): *0-1 times/week*

Beef, red meats

Note -

The following food recommendations are for the generic type. Additionally, you may need from a holistic healer or nutritionist, something more specific for your individuality.

<u>Eat</u>
Deficient Foods

Phosphorus: *1-2 servings/day*

Soda water (unsugared), brewer's yeast, seeds (pumpkin, squash, sunflower, sesame), soybeans, pinto beans, nuts (Brazil, almonds, peanuts, walnuts, cashews, pecans), rye, beef liver, scallops, wheat, cheddar and cottage cheese, barley, oats, eggs, milk, lentils, garlic.

Potassium: *1-2 servings/day*

Dulse, kelp, blackstrap molasses, rice (bran, hulls polish), raisins, parsley, dried prunes, dates, dried figs, avocados, yams, white beans, watercress, alfalfa, tomatoes, rhubarb, avocado, beet greens, Swiss chard, parsnips, halibut, millet, Chinese chestnuts, spinach, baked potato with skin, plain yogurt, salmon, banana,

Calcium, Fluorine: *1-2 servings/day*

Kelp, goat's cheese, raw cabbage, Swiss cheese, turnip greens, parsley, dandelion greens, garlic, raw cauliflower, cabbage, cod liver oil, watercress, tofu, dried figs, yogurt, ripe olives, sauerkraut, spinach, sprouts, watercress, broccoli, spinach, romaine lettuce, dried apricots.

<u>Eat</u>

Nitrogen (vegetable):

Legumes, peas, beans, black-eyed peas, pasta, spirulina, seeds (except pumpkin, sesame, squash, sunflower) — 1-2 servings daily
Eggs, poultry, fish — 3-4 times weekly
Note: Eat any healthy foods you desire, but be sure to include the type foods in your daily choices.

Medeic Nutritional Supplements

- **Multi-Vitamins** —
  [Take all supplements with food]
  2 capsules/day
- **Potassium** —
  99 mg/day
- **Calcium** —
  500 mg. (with magnesium)/twice daily
- **Phosphorus** —
  Obtain Phosfood tabs from a good Health Food Store (best if made by Standard Process Labs: take as directed on the product).
- **Herbs** —
  Brain detox – Chickweed or Valerian Root
  Organ detox – Red Clover or Strawberry Leaf
  (One capsule, twice daily for one month; then one capsule, three times weekly.)
- **Lecithin** —
  1,300 mg/three times weekly
- **Evening Primrose or Flaxseed Oil**
  —1 soft-gel/day

Note: Be sure to take these supplements if you have ill-health. If in good health, take them at least 3-4 times/week.

Important Medeic Health Concerns

Remember that your nervous system genetics require the *Muscle* type Food Guide for health—you may enjoy eating flesh but your health improves as you embrace a semi-vegetarian diet.

► *Rocine: "You should avoid milk, meats, sugar, starches, fatty foods, alcohol, caffeine, stimulating spices and foods. Your greatest need is to join a church in which the people are moral, loving, and religious."*

[This advice from Rocine would surely help you, but it is a tall order with some of you!]

You need vegetable proteins daily and should minimize your animal protein and dairy intake. Dairy allergy is common and calcium should be obtained from green leafy vegetables, citrus fruits and juices.

MEDEIC FOOD GUIDE

Aim for -
50% Proteins, complex carbohydrates
50% Fruits, salads, vegetables

and
50% Raw food diet
50% Cooked foods

Avoid dairy foods and salt!
Re-read Rocine's advice!
Take the recommended supplements.

Medeic Weight Loss

You invariably need to gain weight! But if needing to burn some fat, follow the type instructions, particularly:

- *Stop* eating beef and chloride foods
- *Protein* drink daily, have about 25-30 grams
- *Eat* your body type deficient mineral foods daily
- *Follow* your *Medeic Guide (as above)*
- *Exercise*: your body type requires intense exercise

- *Simple sugars:* stop all white table sugar and high-fructose corn syrup and drinks containing these sugars
- *Hypoglycemia:* this hormonal imbalance stops fat loss, and usually initiates more fat production, so if you have this problem it is vital to deal with it: take *pantothenic acid,* 500 mg/twice daily with food
- *Calories:* As with any dietary approach, calories in, must be *less than* calories out! Most markets sell a calorie booklet; make notes of your daily intake, and in most instances keep it under about 1500 calories/day

———

Muscle Types
General Food Guide
(Carnivores)

Important Note

The Food Guide addresses the <u>Acid-Alkaline</u> aspect of your food intake, along with the <u>Type Mineral</u> factor presented throughout this book. It does <u>not</u> necessarily address calories or other dietary factors that may be pertinent to your personal health needs whether medical or appropriate for some other dietary need. So use your common sense and just include the factors described here with whatever healthy dietary choices you usually make.

For other nutrient information, consult with nutritional books or with holistic nutritional doctors. In this regard, I particularly recommend the advice of Andrew Weil, M.D.

Muscle Types
General Food Guide

(Not for the Nitropheric Type)

This chapter presents a general Food Guide, upon which you superimpose the nutritional information from your type chapter. As a Muscle body type your genetics require flesh foods.

Meat/Flesh Intake

Most muscle types should limit red meat to once or less weekly, while eggs, lamb, fish, or poultry are excellent in moderation. If ill or diseased, be sure to eat daily, one or two servings from each *deficient minerals* list. If not ill, eat them at least three times weekly for health maintenance. If this diet is similar to your present diet, but healing is sluggish, then:

- Decrease your carbohydrate and protein intake by about one-third
- Increase your fruit, salad, and vegetable intake by about one-third
- Consult with a holistic doctor, preferably one versed in nutritional and emotional evaluation

---

Over-Acid or Over-Alkaline?

Just as a log of wood burned in your fireplace leaves a mineral-ash, food ash refers to the minerals remaining after metabolizing foods in your tissues:

- Fruits, vegetables **alkalinize** tissues
- Proteins, carbohydrates **acidify** tissues

Usually You Are Over-Acid Due To:

- Excessive intake of dairy foods
- Excessive intake of proteins and carbohydrates
- Deficient intake of fruits, salads and vegetables
- Accumulated metabolic waste-acids (from years of eating excessive acid-ash foods, meats and carbohydrates, and from lack of exercise)
- You need to estimate the ratio of foods eaten. Generally, eat the following *approximate* ratios for your health:

50% <u>Alkaline-ash</u> foods *(fruits, salads, vegetables)*

50% <u>Acid-ash</u> foods *(complex carbohydrates like starches, grains, cereals, breads, flour products; and proteins)*

Approximate your food ratios. On any particular day, it does not matter if one meal is mostly alkaline, and another mostly acid—just try to balance it out for the day! If you get it wrong, try again tomorrow. It is a subjective call that you make, and it is what you do over weeks, months, or years that make the difference—not on any one or two days.

———

If Vegetarian

As a general indication, if you follow a vegetarian diet substitute vegetable sources of protein for the any flesh in the food guide. Note that contrary to most alkaline-ash vegetarian diets you need something different:

*You need an **acid-ash** vegetarian diet high in complex carbohydrates and vegetable proteins.*

Because of your high need for protein, you usually require a vegetable powdered protein supplement in juice (about 25-30 grams daily).

———

Important

- Minimize white sugar and alcohol intake.
- If desired, interchange lunches for dinners.

- Never eat foods you are allergic to, no matter what I recommend; if allergic, or suspect a food allergy, eliminate it and substitute from your type mineral lists.
- Eat the right foods 80-90% of the time and the Food Guide will work for you; unlike some types you do not have to live out of a health food store (although such foods are healthier for you).

▶ *Omit eating the excessive minerals in your type chapter, and be sure to eat one or two servings from the deficient list daily.*

Finally, in addition to your body type needs, other holistic healing matters also need your attention. I strongly suggest that you refer to my web site and earlier books for that information: *DrStenbeck.net*

———

Acid/Alkaline Genetics Chart

The following chart reflects each Muscle Type and its acid or alkaline-ash food needs. These ratios change if you are unhealthy or over age 45-50. Refer back to your body type and review the *Acid/alkaline* instructions.

———

Acid/Alkaline Genetics, Dietary-Ash, and Raw Food Needs

This chart shows the Rocine types, their acid or alkaline food needs, and the percentage of raw foods needed for your health and healing.

- Apply your Type Minerals to the Food Guide

Type	Acid/Alkaline Genetics	% Food-Ash Needed	% Raw Food Needed
Calciferic	Alkaline	70% acid	30
Carbogenic	Alkaline	50-50	50
Desmogenic	Alkaline	70% acid	50
Eldic	Intermediate	50-50	50
Medeic	Intermediate	50-50	50
Myogenic	Intermediate	50-50	50
Nervimotive	Alkaline	70% acid	50
Nitropheric	Acid	70% alkaline	70
Pallinomic	Alkaline	50-50	30

The above percentages vary depending on aging and the health of individual types.

Muscle Types / Food Guide
Breakfast

[Superimpose the nutritional information from your

EGGS (1-2) with lettuce, tomato, or salad, whole grain toast; (add bacon or sausage 1-3 times weekly if desired)*
— 2-4 times/ week; or

FRUIT fresh salad, and protein (yogurt, milk, cheeses, seeds, nuts)
—1-3 times/ week; or

CEREALS, with fruit, seeds, nuts
—2-5 times/ week; or

OTHER choices
— 0-1 times weekly

Daily liquids:
Pure water, citrus, vegetable juices, soups, other — as desired
Coffee, teas —0-2 cups

[Include selections from your type mineral needs everyday.]

Muscle Types / Food Guide

<u>Lunch</u>

SALADS, mixed green, protein (poultry, fish, egg, cheese, seeds or nuts, etc.), whole grain breads
 [Dressing: olive oil/ vinegar; low-fat, low-cal dressings]
— 2-4 times/ week; or

SANDWICH, whole grains with a protein (cheese, tuna, ham, etc.); and salad and/ or vegetables
— 1-4 times/ week; or

POULTRY, FISH, 3-6 oz., with a mixed green salad and/ or vegetables
—1-3 times/ week; or

OTHER choices (with salad or vegetables)
—1-2 times/ week

[Other oils permitted, but less ideal is soybean oil, a common allergen; minimize commercial dressings. Be sure to include two or more selections from your type food lists in your daily food intake. For in-between meal snacks, eat fruit or vegetables with seeds/ nuts.]

[Include selections from your type mineral needs everyday.]

Muscle Types / Food Guide
<u>Dinner</u>

POULTRY, FISH *(4-6 oz.), with salad and/ or vegetables*
—2-4 times/ week; or

PASTA with protein (chicken, etc.) with salad and/ or vegetables
— 2-4 times/ week; or

VEGETARIAN meal with salad and/ or vegetables
—1-3 times/ week; or

LEAN BEEF (4-6 oz.) with salad and/ or vegetables
— 0-1 times/ week

OTHER choices with salad and/ or vegetables
— 0-1 times/ week

<u>Desserts:</u>
Fruits, fresh — as desired
Low-sugar, healthy desserts
— 0-3 times/ wk

[Include selections from your type mineral needs everyday.]

Food Guide Notes

Steamed Vegetables —

Minerals are lost in the boiling of vegetables; steaming or wok cooking is best.

Food Combinations —

If you have a weak digestive system then eating proteins at the same meal with starches often results in indigestion, gas, or constipation.

Periodic Detox —

You tend to over-indulge in acid-ash foods (proteins and carbohydrates), and often need occasional elimination diets for tissue waste-acid removal. Have a holistic doctor or nutritionist supervise such detox (where you have an alkaline-ash diet along with protein supplementation).

Minimize —

- Fatty foods
- Commercial salad dressings
- Beef, red meats, processed meats
- Coffee, white sugar, corn syrup, alcohol

Vegetarian Proteins —

You require a carnivorous diet. An exception is the *nitropheric* type who functions best with a *vegetarian* diet. The other muscle types are born to be carnivores. It is very difficult for the other muscle types to be pure vegetarians because of their strong intuitive cravings for fish, poultry, meat, or eggs. If you are vegetarian, then because of your high needs for amino acids and acid-ash foods, you should take a protein supplement of 30-40 grams/day (powdered protein in juice).

Healthy Weight —

Several of you gain weight as the ravages of age, lack of exercise and dietary excesses take their toll. By eating according to your body type, you should naturally lose excess weight. Each type also has a few individual factors that only apply to them!

You have a good ability to lose weight by following the Food Guide instructions. The most common problem I find with your weight-control is liver and kidney irritation due to food allergies, which results in extra pounds. The key is to eat non-allergic foods.

If drinking more than 3-4 cups daily of coffee or tea, you may have a hypoglycemic problem (low blood sugar), which contributes to making fat, ill-health, and delayed healing. (Refer to the earlier books for help with this healing.)

―――

Appendix

Brief Extracts from
<u>The 22 Unique Body Types 68</u>

Appendix A

Types
(Brief extract)

Type comes from 'typus' meaning an image or impression, the study of types being called typology.

▶ *Rocine: "A combination of mental and structural features is consistently found in people of the same type."*

Rocine wrote that all types are a mixture of positive and negative qualities. He based his work on the biochemical individuality of our *mineral* absorption and utilization. Of course, all minerals are absorbed, but he postulated that different types of people *selectively* absorb certain minerals, to a greater or lesser extent, requiring specific mineral foods for their enhanced health and healing.

▶ *The type information cannot predict what or who you will become, or how successful or not, but your type is capable of bringing a creative excellence to whatever you do in life. If your type has negative qualities that you disagree with, remember that they are only tendencies and may or may not manifest in you.*

This book enlarges on Rocine's premise (early 1900's), integrated with the later research of Herbert Sheldon, M.D., Ph.D., at Harvard University (1930's), along with my fifty years of observations and experience with this subject.

Comparing your shared physical (and sometimes psychological) descriptions with the Celebrity Lists further assists the identification of your type. It is not that you will look exactly like, or be a twin to, any particular celebrity. Look closely at a celebrity's features: face, profile, height, weight, head, etc. If you know something about their talents, beliefs, success and failure spheres, health and weight challenges, attitudes and behaviors, etc., then you get clues as to what your type may be.

Understanding Types and Sub-Types

Each of us has a clearly discernible dominant type. Visualize the celebrity examples from movies, politics, sports, the arts and public life, and try to identify with their physical features. Look for similar features, remembering that you will not recognize all attributes in yourself. You are not looking for your twin!

The sub-type issue is the main reason people of the same major type can look so different. Remember that a type description does not characterize you exactly, but depicts your individual variant of a type.

▶ *The type questionnaire pinpoints the major features of that type: if the celebrity examples are unhelpful, you may be an unusual variant (in which case ignore the celebrity issue and give yourself 7 points on Question 1).*

———

Minerals

Minerals are essential life nutrients that accelerate enzyme and chemical reactions and provide a basis for your body typing. Although found in all tissues, different minerals tend to be concentrated in certain organs, their presence or absence contributing to the healing of such tissues; e.g., zinc accelerates prostate healing; calcium and manganese promote bone, joint and connective tissue healing.

Specific foods nurture each type, some people needing meats for their health others needing a vegetarian diet. A high potassium diet nurtures one person, while another needs high sulfur, calcium, zinc, or another mineral.

Mineral Digestion and Absorption

Compared to vitamins, minerals are *difficult* to digest, absorb, and utilize. In people with strong digestive systems, this aspect may not be important. The following factors should be in place for optimal mineral metabolism:

1. Stomach Hydrochloric Acid Production
2. Parathyroid Hormone Balance
3. Organ Toxic Metal and Chemical Removal
    [See details in <u>The 22 Unique Body Types</u>.]

———

Total Body Healing

Note that from a holistic healing perspective, in addition to minerals and type information, the following healing factors are necessary:

> *Nutrient Balance*
> *Mental Balance*
> *Emotional Balance*
> *Spiritual Balance*
> *Detoxifying Integrity*

The above factors are all important to your total healing especially if you are interested in self-healing (see my earlier books).

———

Appendix B

Researchers
(Brief extract)

The predominant workers in this area of human individuality from around 1880's to the 1960's are Herbert Sheldon, M.D., Ph.D., Roger Williams, Ph.D., and Victor Rocine, D.Sc.

Much information on Sheldon's research exists on-line and in medical psychology libraries; for interested readers there are other lines of research published in the last century. This present book is primarily about Rocine's body types.

Herbert Sheldon M.D., Ph.D.

In contrast to Rocine, Sheldon at Harvard University in the 1930's was trained in the scientific method and did painstaking research and publishing on human individuality. In comparing his findings with Rocine's work, a direct putative correlation is visible.

Roger J. Williams, Ph.D.

Another significant researcher in human individuality is the renowned scientist and biochemist, Roger J. Williams. He demonstrated that different people have varying levels of nutrients, enzymes, and other metabolic chemicals in their bloodstreams.

▶ *Williams's research firmly expands on the premise of individual nutritional needs in human beings. If interested in his research, I highly recommend his book Biochemial Individuality.*

Victor Rocine, D.Sc.

Note that when a negative feature is indicated, say neurotic tendencies, all members of the type are <u>not</u> that way; it is a type tendency reported by Rocine.

Rocine studied type-related diseases finding links between mineral and dietary factors with individual types and their diseases. In each body type, one or more dominant minerals are preferentially absorbed and utilized over other minerals.

He recognized discrete body types from their physical appearance finding genetically based mineral dominance to be the determining feature. He also correlated their physical features with psychological characteristics.

———

Genetics, Types, and Diet
(Brief extract)

This section deals with how nervous system genetics helps determine your eating choices for health: you are either born to be a predominant meat eater, a partial or complete vegetarian, or something between the two. The genetic factor determining this dietary aspect is the *sympathetic and parasympathetic* components of your central nervous system. This represents a basic factor in eating for health.

This chapter helps you understand your dietary inheritance, although instinctively, you may already have arrived there!

- If born **sympathetic** dominant you are *genetically acid*, desiring a predominantly *vegetarian* diet for your health (about 70% fruit, salad, vegetables to 30% proteins and carbohydrates).

- If born **parasympathetic** dominant you are *genetically alkaline*, desiring a predominantly *carnivorous* diet for your health (about 70% proteins, carbohydrates to 30% fruits, salads, vegetables). Few of you ever choose to become vegetarian because of the difficulty in satisfying your protein needs without meats.

- If born ***intermediate*** dominant you may eat food groups with little concern for the acid/alkaline factor. However, after age 40, you need a semi-vegetarian diet for healthy eating.

———

Chart of Relative Nervous System Dominance

In the following Chart, if you relate to many of the symptoms on one side you probably have that nervous system dominance; relating to both sides indicates *Intermediate* dominance.

If Vegetarian (Over-acid) --
> *Eat 70% fruits, salads, vegetables*
> *And 30% proteins, carbohydrates*

If Carnivore (Over-alkaline) --
> *Eat 70% proteins, carbohydrates*
> *And 30% fruits, salads, vegetables*

If Intermediate --
> *Eat 50:50 of acid and alkaline-ash foods*

Make an *approximate* estimate of your daily acid and alkaline food intake (such ratios varying from type to type).

———

Symptoms of Relative
Genetic Dominance

Vegetarians (Over-acid)	Carnivores (Over-alkaline)
Sympathetic Dominance	*Parasympathetic Dominance*
little or no flesh desire	desire flesh
easily constipated	rarely constipated
slow digestion	fast digestion
easily dehydrated	not dehydrated
strong thirst	low thirst
pale face	flushed face
high pulse after food	slow pulse after food
easy gag reflex	slow gag reflex
cool dry skin	moist warm skin
nervous stomach	calm stomach
little eyelid blinking	much blinking
nervous tendency	mostly calm
slower healing	faster healing
low oxygen-uptake	good oxygen-uptake
easily breathless	seldom breathless
insomnia common	sleep easier
few muscle cramps	some night cramps
calcium deposits rare	get calcium deposits

Appendix D

Help Identifying your Body Type with Dr. Stenbeck

If you desire help in identifying your body type, follow these instructions, and answer the questionnaire. For further information and fees, send me an email from page one of the website:

DrStenbeck.net

First name: _______________________

Country of birth: _______________________

Upload photos and send to the above website:

- Head and shoulders: front and side views

- Full body: front and side views

- Also 1-2 teenage views

- If possible, casual photos of mother, father, siblings

MY TYPE CLASS MAY BE: _______________

   (Thin, Muscle, or Fat)

AGE   -   _________

HEIGHT   -   _________ feet/inches

MY WEIGHT -   _________ pounds

   Heaviest at age: _________

- Lightest as adult: __________

- Estimate age 15: __________

VISION - Excellent Average   Poor:

HAIR - Natural color: __________

- Thin/thick?   __________

- balding?   __________

SKIN - Quality: __________

- History of acne, boils, other:

____

____

TEETH   - Strong   Weak   Dentures

- Cavity history: Many   Moderate Few

MUSCLES - Strong   Average   Weak

Sports played __________________________

JOINTS   - Strong   Average   Weak

HEALTH - Childhood diseases?

____

____

- Adult diseases?

____

AVERAGE DIET

- Beef   ___________ (times/week)

  - Poultry   ___________ (times/week)

  - Fish   ___________ (times/week)

  - Eggs   ___________ (times/week)

  - Water   ___________ (glasses/day):

  - Vegetarian? Vegan?   ___________

  - Other?   _____________________

  - Did your childhood diet differ? _______

The above will help me know who you are! I will send you a follow-up questionnaire for further help in identifying your body type.

Appendix E

On-line Health Consultation
with Dr. Stenbeck

For further information, or to comment on this book, or to receive a response on any health issue from a holistic viewpoint, send an email inquiry from page one of my website:

DrStenbeck.net

Following that, I will suggest further healing needs, which we may pursue with an on-line consult.

———

Appendix F

Notes

See my book *The 22 Unique Body Types,* available at the usual online source, for further information and details on all of the 22 Types. The Appendix in that book has further information about:

Mineral Functions and Food Sources

Further Reading

———